BREAST CANCER

Current and Emerging Trends in Detection and Treatment

TERRY L. SMITH

The Rosen Publishing Group, Inc., New York

Published in 2006 by The Rosen Publishing Group, Inc.
29 East 21st Street, New York, NY 10010

Copyright © 2006 by The Rosen Publishing Group, Inc.

First Edition

Library of Congress Cataloging-in-Publication Data

Smith, Terry L.
Breast cancer: current and emerging trends in detection and treatment / Terry L. Smith.
    p. cm.—(Cancer and modern science)
Includes bibliographical references and index.
ISBN 1-4042-0386-9 (lib. bdg.)
1. Breast—Cancer.
I. Title. II. Series.
RC280.B8S56 2006
616.99'449—dc22

                                               2005000130

Manufactured in Malaysia

On the cover: Electron micrograph of two breast cancer cells entering the final stage of division.

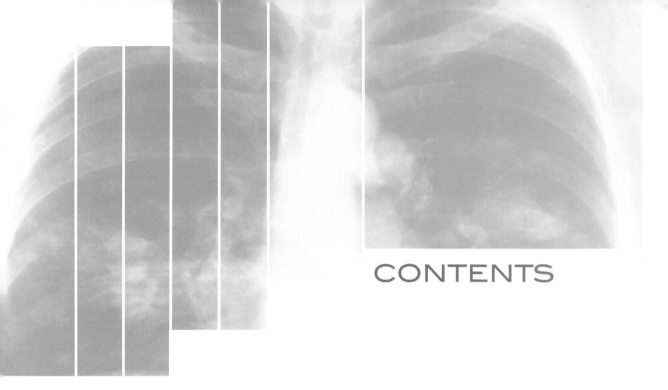

CONTENTS

INTRODUCTION

A hardy band of scientists and support personnel huddled under a 165-foot-wide (50-meter-wide) dome at the South Pole. The date was March 21, 1999, and an Antarctic storm obscured their view of the setting Sun. The Sun would not rise again over the South Pole until September. Surrounded by darkness and ice, the "Polies" were well prepared for the long winter, or so they thought. During this time, their only contact with the rest of the world would be through the Internet and limited use of a satellite phone. Indeed, the cold weather, with temperatures that could fall to −100°F (−73°C), would make landing an airplane impossible.

At this remote location, astronomers, meteorologists, and physicists would carry out scientific experiments for the National Science Foundation. Meanwhile, a skilled group of computer technicians, mechanics, cooks, and others were responsible for the heating, cooking, and other support systems upon which their very lives depended. Dr. Jerri Nielsen was a forty-six-year-old emergency room physician from Ohio. Serving

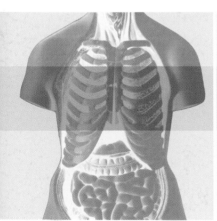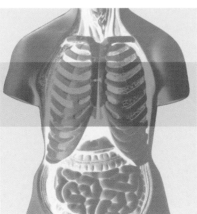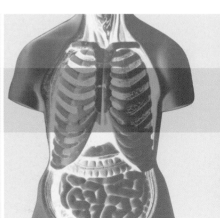

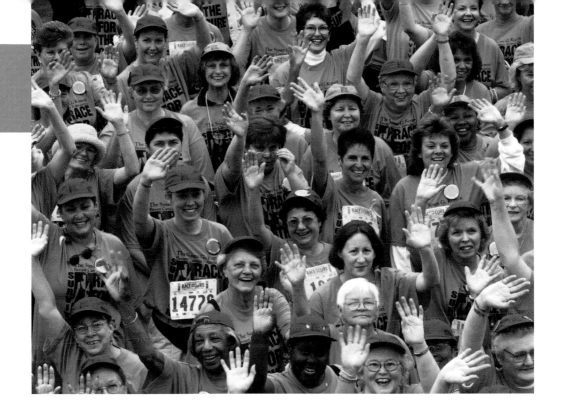

Breast cancer survivors in St. Louis, Missouri, wave to the cameras before starting a walk to raise money for breast cancer research. This was an event of the Susan G. Komen Foundation, founded by Nancy Brinker in memory of her sister who died of breast cancer in the early 1980s, when there was little public awareness of the disease. This foundation's mission is to promote breast cancer education and awareness, provide patient support, and raise money for research.

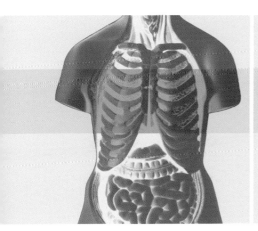

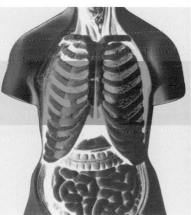

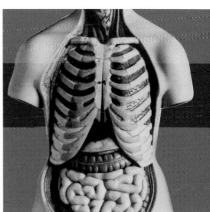

as the group's doctor, she was responsible for any medical needs that might arise among the "winter-over" crew of forty-one men and women. Respiratory infections, frostbite, and injuries occupied most of her time. She also had to be prepared to handle dental emergencies, mental health issues, and any serious illnesses that might arise, using only the limited provisions in her small medical clinic. Little did Dr. Nielsen know that she herself would soon become her biggest medical challenge. Around the time the Sun went down, she discovered a lump in her breast.

Dr. Nielsen had undergone a thorough medical examination just a few months earlier. This exam included a mammogram that was reported as normal. So when she first discovered the lump, she drew the same conclusion that she probably would have drawn had she been at home—that the lump was associated with her menstrual cycle and would soon disappear. Yet a month later, instead of the hoped-for disappearance, Dr. Nielsen found that the lump was even larger. Back home in the United States, this finding would have led to a series of diagnostic tests and appropriate follow-up treatments, all conducted by physicians specializing in breast cancer. Isolated at the South Pole, Dr. Nielsen set out to diagnose the lump as best she could, using only her limited supplies and consulting with U.S. physicians via the Internet.

A carpenter with some veterinary experience was selected to assist her in performing a biopsy, which consisted of injecting a needle into the lump and withdrawing a small amount of tissue. Dr. Nielsen had him practice first on potatoes and apples. Ice, in abundant supply at the South Pole, served as a local anesthetic. The extracted tissue was prepared on slides, and images were e-mailed to cancer specialists in the United States to be viewed under a microscope. However, the process proved inadequate for diagnosis, leaving Dr. Nielsen in emotional turmoil and her physicians in the United States puzzled over how to proceed with her care. Finally, as the lump continued to grow, Dr. Nielsen's physicians suspected that it was cancer, even without

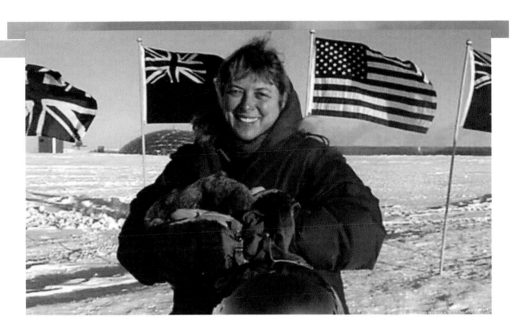

Dr. Jerri Nielsen is pictured here on October 7, 1999 at the South Pole. Dr. Nielsen had had a history of benign breast cysts. Before leaving for the South Pole, she underwent an extensive physical examination that included a mammogram. Nevertheless, she was diagnosed with breast cancer during her stay on the South Pole. After returning to the United States and undergoing treatment, she was cancer free by April 2000.

biopsy proof. An Air Force emergency airdrop of medical supplies was soon arranged. News reports in the United States had the nation waiting anxiously to learn the fate of the doctor at the South Pole who had become her own patient.

The airdrop included cancer chemotherapy and equipment for video transmissions. Once the emergency supplies were successfully dropped and retrieved by the winter-over crew, Dr. Nielsen transmitted images from a second biopsy. At that stage, the breast cancer diagnosis was confirmed. Weekly chemotherapy sessions, with assistance from fellow Polies and instructions from physicians linked by the new video equipment, were begun immediately when the diagnosis was established. Dr. Nielsen did not escape the feelings of nausea, fatigue, and other side effects that accompany chemotherapy. Yet, as the only resident physician, she managed to maintain her regular clinic appointments to care for the other Polies. On October 16, in the midst of springtime storms, Dr. Nielsen was "extracted" early from the Pole and flown to the United States, where she met the doctors she had only seen on video during her chemotherapy sessions. She was switched to a conventional breast cancer treatment program and found to be free of detectable cancer after her treatment.

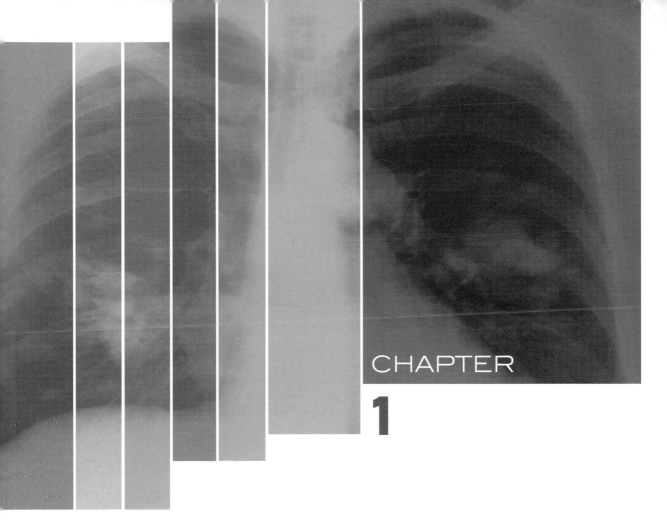

BREAST CANCER THROUGHOUT HISTORY

Black bile, *karkinos*, nun's disease, God's punishment—whatever name was used, women throughout the ages have known and feared breast cancer. Long ago, breast cancer was the most recognized form of cancer. Though other forms of cancer occurred, these tumors were hidden from sight, and a patient would die with no one knowing the cause. Breast cancer, however, was a very visible disease, producing lumps on a private part of a woman's body. Such lumps grew and grew until they eventually broke through the skin and gave off a foul-smelling black discharge. A woman who discovered a lump in her breast knew she might soon die a horrible death. But just like today, most women throughout history who discovered lumps in their breasts did not have cancer.

The Greek physician Hippocrates (c. 460–377 BC) made a careful study of the causes of human diseases. He believed that the body contained four fluids—blood, phlegm, yellow bile, and black bile—all of which needed to be in proper balance or disease would occur. Because advanced breast tumors had a dark color and gave off a black fluid when they grew large, he concluded that the disease was caused by an excess of black bile in a woman's body. This belief led Greek physicians to treat breast cancer by ridding the body of the excess bile, using methods such as bleedings or administering medicines that would make a woman vomit. The theory that breast cancer was caused by an imbalance in body fluids persisted for many centuries.

RISE OF SURGERY TO TREAT BREAST CANCER

By the 1700s, physicians had learned little more about the causes of breast cancer. However, they gradually became convinced that the way to treat it was to remove the diseased breast. Surgeons devised elaborate tools and procedures for cutting away the breast, even before the time of sterile operating rooms and anesthesia. They promised to cure women of their disease, if only they would undergo the painful and disfiguring surgery.

During the nineteenth century and into the twentieth century, surgeons remained convinced that breast cancer was a local disease that they could cure, if only they cut away enough of the tumor and if women would come for surgery as soon as a lump was noted. Fortunately for the women involved, several discoveries helped them endure treatment with less pain and increase their chances of survival. These included the discovery of ether for anesthesia (the temporary

DR. WILLIAM HALSTED AND THE RADICAL MASTECTOMY

At the beginning of the twentieth century, Dr. William Halsted of Johns Hopkins University Medical School was an internationally recognized surgeon, known for his pioneering surgical techniques, the training of young surgeons, and the invention of the rubber surgical glove. He had a special interest in breast cancer and traveled the world to study how it could best be treated. Dr. Halsted became convinced that breast cancer could be cured by surgery and that the surgery must be extensive, removing not only the breast but the underlying chest muscle and the nodes in the armpit. The procedure was called a "radical" mastectomy, and it became the standard treatment for breast cancer for the next fifty years.

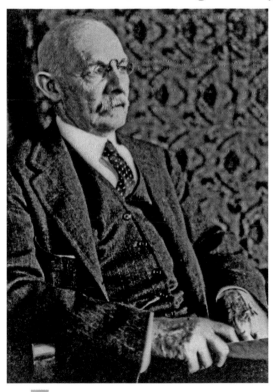

American surgeon Dr. William Halstead (1852–1922) believed that the more aggressive the surgery, the better the patient's chance for survival. Many patients who underwent the disfiguring surgery later developed metastases of breast cancer in other distant sites, and eventually succumbed to cancer.

This is an X-ray, frontal view, showing a metastasis of breast cancer in the right humerus. (See arrow pointing to the white lesion marked with holes.) Although any cancer can spread to the bone, bony metastases are most common in breast cancer. Besides proximal long bones, breast cancer, if it spreads to bone, affects the pelvis, spine, and ribs.

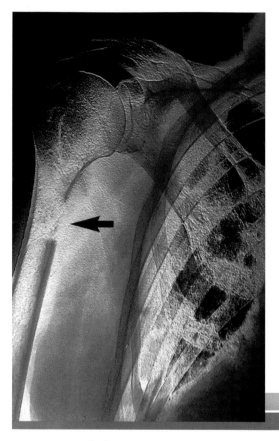

loss of the sensation of pain), the discovery of the importance of sterile instruments and operating rooms to reduce the chance of infection, and finally the discovery of antibiotics in case infection occurred. When microscopes became available and the cellular structures of plants and animals were recognized, the science of pathology came into being. For the first time, physicians were able to study cells from a breast lump under a microscope and decide if they were cancerous. From then on, only those women who truly had cancer required the disfiguring surgery that came to be known as mastectomy.

DISCOVERY OF OTHER EFFECTIVE TREATMENTS

The scientific advances made during World War II (1939–1945) increased Americans' hopes that scientists could also find a cure for cancer. Some

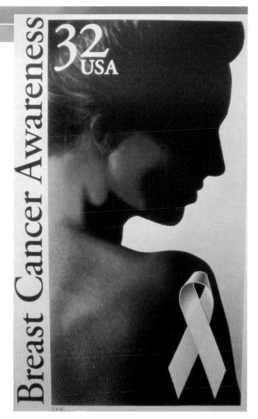

According to the American Cancer Society, 211,240 women will get breast cancer in 2005. However, because of aggressive awareness campaigns that stress the importance of self-examinations and mammograms, these women have an increased rate of survival. The United States Postal Service even joined the campaign when they issued this postal stamp in 1996.

medical researchers began to question the theory that breast cancer was a local disease curable by surgery. They claimed that cancer cells could spread throughout the body by the blood and lymph systems, and no amount of surgery would cure a woman if these cells had spread. At the same time, drugs were discovered that could kill cancer cells. Treating cancer with drugs was then tested.

Scientists also discovered that cancer cells could be killed with radiotherapy. Large clinical trials—in which the treatments for thousands of women with breast cancer were decided by a process of randomization (similar to the flip of a coin)—allowed the scientists to prove that surgery was not sufficient treatment. These clinical trials also proved that it was not always necessary for surgeons to remove the entire breast and that radiotherapy and chemotherapy were also essential. Modern science finally proved what the ancient Greeks had concluded—that breast cancer is a disease of the whole body and must be treated accordingly.

ROLE OF WOMEN IN TREATMENT ADVANCES

While scientists were working to prove that such radical breast cancer surgery was not always required, women were busy raising the issue with the public. Women of earlier times had been too embarrassed to let others know they had breast cancer, and there was little public discussion of the disease. Gradually, the disease came "out of the closet" beginning in the 1970s. Child actress Shirley Temple Black and First Lady Betty Ford openly discussed their diagnoses of breast cancer in the public media. The accompanying rise of feminism encouraged women to take charge of their own bodies and to question the treatment decisions of the male-dominated medical establishment. More young women trained as physicians and scientists. Women whose lives were affected by breast cancer began to organize and form groups to help other women with the disease. They began to lobby the government for more breast cancer research funding. A woman diagnosed with breast cancer today knows that she joins a huge sisterhood of cancer survivors ready to help her along the way to recovery.

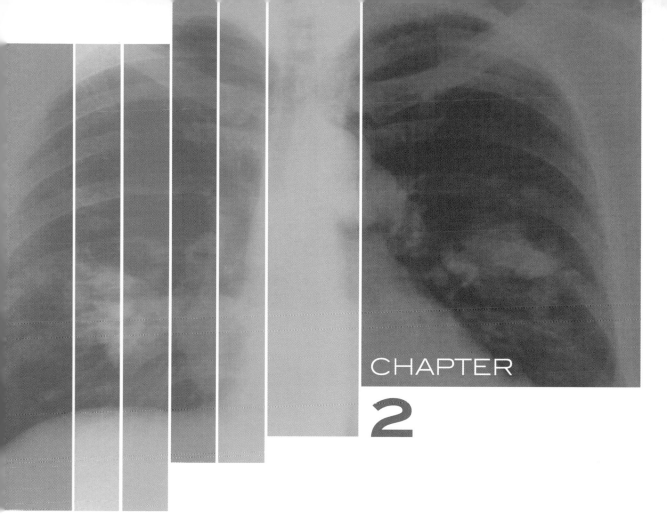

WHAT IS BREAST CANCER?

Mammary glands—breasts—are what define us as mammals. Breasts are part of a woman's reproductive system. Their main purpose is to produce milk for feeding an infant after a female gives birth. Breasts come in a wide range of sizes and shapes, all of which are perfectly normal as long as they can produce milk. Breast tissue extends beyond the visible breast, from the collarbone down to near the bottom of the ribs. Chest muscles lie between breast tissue and the ribs.

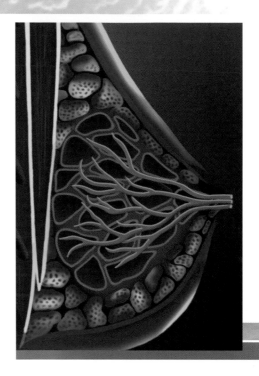

This diagram of the breast shows the lobes of the breast (dark red), where milk is produced, surrounded by fatty tissue. The lactiferous ducts (purple) lead from the lobes to the nipple and carry milk there when a woman is breast-feeding. Each breast has between five and ten ductal systems, each with its own opening at the nipple. The pectoral muscle in the chest wall, upon which the breasts lie, is also depicted. Besides these components, the breast is made up of nerves, veins, arteries, and connective tissue.

Each breast consists of fifteen to twenty lobes that are arranged like spokes on a wheel around the central nipple, which is the small tip of the breast. A lobe is made up of many smaller lobes, or lobules, which contain groups of tiny glands that can produce milk. Small tubes, or ducts, lead from these lobules to the nipple, which is how milk reaches the nipple when a woman is nursing an infant. Fat tissue surrounds the lobes and ducts, and makes up about a third of breast tissue.

Breasts also contain nerves, blood vessels, lymph vessels, and some tissues necessary for support. The lymph vessels play an important role in conducting fluids from the cells of breast tissues to small organs called lymph nodes, which are located in several areas surrounding the breasts. Most of the lymph nodes near the breast are located in the area under a woman's arm, also referred to as the axilla. Lymph nodes serve as filters for the body's fluids, and they are able to signal the immune system to launch an attack if they detect harmful substances. We can think of them as the body's garbage collectors.

BREAST CANCER IS A DISEASE OF GENES

All breast cancers result from an alteration of the normal genetic process. The problem scientists have in learning how to prevent or cure breast cancer is that the genetic process is so complicated, and there are so many different things that can go wrong that lead to cancer.

Using the information coded in a single gene, a cell can produce a protein that acts to carry out the needed function. For example, there is a gene that becomes active when a young woman reaches puberty. Its purpose is to produce a protein that causes her breasts to grow. Thousands of such genes are linked together into the chromosomes found in the nucleus of every human cell.

For breast cancer to develop, a series of mutations, or flaws, must take place within the genetic material of a breast cell. These mutations may be inherited flaws in certain genes, or they may result from environmental influences or an error that occurs by chance. Each

continued on page 18

Above is a colored electron micrograph of ductal carcinoma, the most common form of breast cancer. The mammary duct is colored red, and the cancer cells are colored pink. The cancer cells are tested for HER-2 overexpression and other tumor markers.

continued from page 17

time a cell divides into two cells, the genetic material must duplicate itself. It is during this process that a mutation in the coded information may occur.

One such alteration that scientists know is related to breast cancer is in the gene they have named HER-2 (for human epidermal growth factor receptor 2). Cells from a newly diagnosed breast tumor are tested to find out if the HER-2 gene is active. This information, combined with information on the size of tumor, whether there are breast cancer cells in nearby nodes, and whether hormone receptors are present, helps a woman and her doctor decide which treatment is best against her tumor.

Along with the breasts, the female reproductive system also includes two ovaries, which are small organs located within the abdomen. In addition to their important role as a place where eggs are stored prior to monthly ovulation, the ovaries produce a hormone called estrogen. Hormones are chemical substances produced within the body and released into the bloodstream, where they travel to other organs in order to control various body functions. Estrogen is a sex hormone and acts specifically to control functions within the breasts and other parts of the female reproductive system. Cells in breast tissue contain tiny structures called estrogen receptors, to which an estrogen molecule can bind and affect the activity of the cell. It is by way of these hormone messengers that the breasts know, for example, to begin the production of milk after a woman has given birth. These hormone receptors also play an important role in cell growth if a woman should develop a cancer in her breast, as we will see in chapter 4.

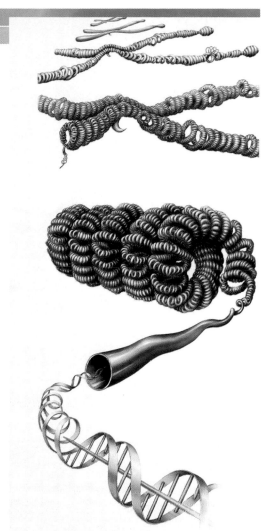

This illustration depicts the makeup of chromosomes. Each chromosome contains many genes, which are in turn made up of sequences of four chemical bases—adenine, thymine, cytosine, and guanine. As seen in the foreground, these bases are incorporated into a double helix structure. Their sequence determines what protein the gene will produce.

THE CANCER PROCESS

All cells in the body, including those that make up the breasts, contain tiny threadlike structures called chromosomes. The chromosomes are made up of thousands of genes that control cell activities. The coordinated actions of cells throughout the body allow us to function as healthy beings. Cells also contain "switches," which are complex biochemical processes designed to switch certain genes to the "on" or "off" position, depending on the role required of a particular cell. If these switches and genes malfunction, then a cell no longer behaves normally. This rarely happens; in most cases, the body's built-in checking system notices that a certain cell is not behaving correctly and acts to protect the body by killing the bad cell.

Yet once in a while, these systems fail to work properly. Mutations in a gene may cause new cells to form when they are not needed, and old

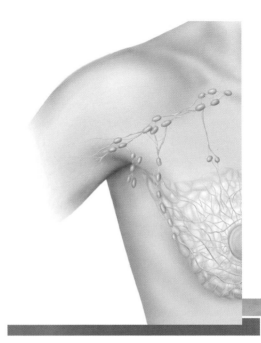

This is an illustration of the chain of lymph nodes of the female breast extending from the axillary nodes of the underarm (examination of which is most important in determining if breast cancer has spread) to the infraclavicular nodes and supraclavicular nodes at and above the collarbone. Most lymph fluid from the breast is first received by the axillary lymph nodes. These nodes then send fluid to the lymph nodes located farther up the chain.

cells may not die when they should. This can lead to a growing clump of cells that eventually make a mass of tissue. In some cases, this mass, or tumor, grows uncontrollably and invades other body tissues, becoming cancer. When such uncontrolled growth occurs among cells in the breast, it is called breast cancer.

Cancer cells may travel through the bloodstream or the lymph system to other parts of the body. If a cancer cell begins to grow at another site in the body, this new growth is called a metastasis of the cancer. Researchers are still trying to understand how this process of metastasis takes place and why breast cancer cells can grow at some sites of the body and not others. For example, the bones, lungs, and liver are sites at which breast cancer cells may grow. Not only must the cancer cells travel to reach these other body sites, but once they get there, conditions must be just right for their growth. Sometimes these cells may remain there without growing for many years, which explains why a cancer metastasis may develop many years after the original cancer has developed. Growths consisting of breast cancer cells in other parts of the body are still referred to as breast cancer, even though they are not in the breast. When cells from these growths are examined under a microscope, they look the same as breast cancer cells.

STAGES OF BREAST CANCER

A tumor growth within the breast is called a primary tumor, while tumors that have spread from the breast to distant sites are called secondary tumors, or metastases. Many breast cancers never spread to distant sites. Doctors classify primary tumors according to their characteristics when they are first detected. Tumors detected before cells have invaded other tissue or when they are very small are regarded as early stage cancer (stage 0 or stage I). Women with these tumors have a very good prognosis, or outcome. Most women with stage 0 or stage I disease are cured of breast cancer following their initial treatment. If the tumor is large or if cancer cells are detected in the lymph nodes of the axilla or other nearby tissues, the cancer is a higher stage (stage II or stage III), and prognosis is not as good for women with these tumors. If a cancer has spread to sites other than the breast area, it is stage IV or metastatic cancer. Although women with stage IV cancers may live for many years, most eventually die from their disease. This is why doctors regard treatment of the primary cancer as so important, which we will learn more about in chapter 4. If spread of the cancer to distant sites can be prevented, a woman is usually cured of breast cancer.

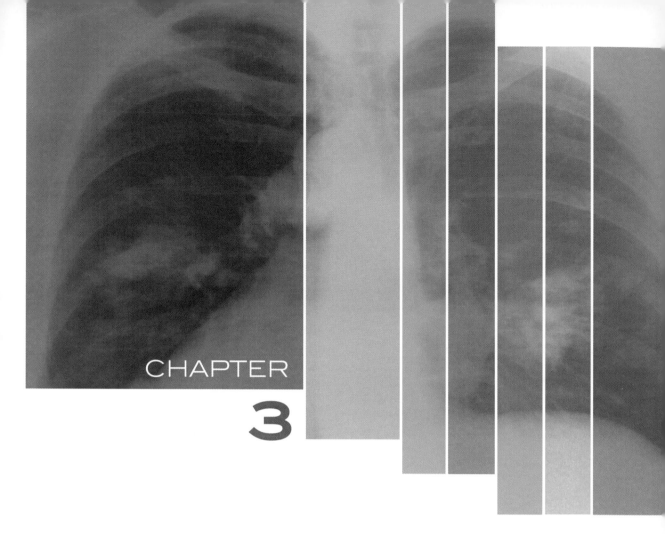

CHAPTER 3

WHO GETS BREAST CANCER?

If a friend or family member of yours has breast cancer, it may begin to seem that breast cancer is a common disease. You will notice that newspapers and magazines often feature stories about prominent women who have breast cancer. You may hear scary statistics, for example, one in eight women will develop breast cancer. Though this statistic is true over the lifetime of a woman, the fact is that breast cancer is a very uncommon disease in young women. It is only during older age that a woman is at substantially increased risk of developing the disease. Age is the most important factor

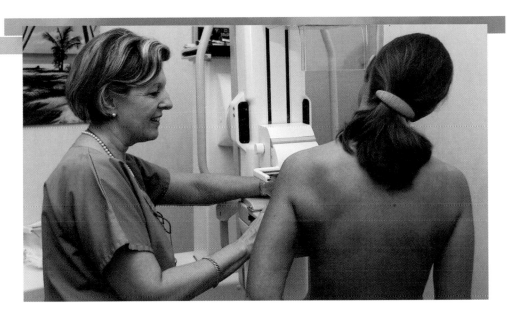

Here, a woman is undergoing a routine mammography examination, assisted by a technician. The duration of the procedure is about fifteen minutes. Each breast is flattened between two plates and then an X-ray image is made. Radiologists who specialize in reading mammograms then look for any lesions or tumors that may exist deep inside the breast tissue and which may not be felt by physical examination alone.

determining a woman's risk of breast cancer. And of those women who do get breast cancer, far more than half of them make a total recovery and continue to live normal lives.

THE CHANGING RISK OF BREAST CANCER

More than 200,000 women in the United States are diagnosed with breast cancer each year, and approximately 40,000 die from the disease. For comparison, a similar number of people die each year in traffic accidents. From 1940 to the early 1980s, breast cancer incidence in the

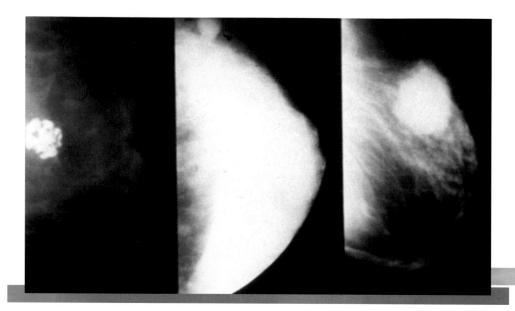

Three types of breast irregularities can appear on a mammogram. Calcium deposits (left) or an area of increased thickening may be a sign of early cancer. Benign tumors, such as the one seen at the top of the center image, are commonly very defined and round. The less compact white spot in the image far right is a malignant tumor.

United States increased by less than 1 percent each year (when adjusted for age of the female population). Scientists believe these increases were due to changes in women's lifestyles, particularly the trend for women to have fewer children. In the 1980s, breast cancer incidence increased at a more rapid pace, about 3 to 4 percent per year, chiefly because a method for detecting breast cancer with X-rays, called mammography, became widely available.

Prior to the use of mammography, some of these cancers diagnosed at a very early stage might never have been detected. Fortunately, despite this trend for an increase in the number of women diagnosed with breast cancer, the age-adjusted rate of deaths from breast cancer has dropped.

Researchers attribute this improvement in breast cancer survival to earlier detection of cancer due to mammography, and to improvements in treatment. Despite this progress, breast cancer remains a serious problem and is the second leading cause of cancer deaths among women after lung cancer.

As we learned in chapter 2, breast cancer occurs due to changes, or mutations, in the genetic material of breast cells that cause the cells to grow out of control. It is not possible to know the causes of these changes in a particular woman who develops breast cancer. However, about 5 to 10 percent of breast cancer cases are explained by certain inherited genetic defects that scientists have named BRCA1 and BRCA2. Researchers have learned that certain women are more likely to have these genetic defects. For example, if a mother or sister has developed breast cancer at a young age, these women have a higher risk of getting breast cancer. A test can determine if a woman carries these inherited defects. Doctors may recommend this test for some young women after discussing with them the number of cancers among family members.

FACTORS ASSOCIATED WITH THE OCCURRENCE OF BREAST CANCER

The development of a breast cancer case is a complex process that involves multiple steps, and may be influenced by many things happening in a woman's body. Breast cancer cells present during early breast development and cells undergoing rapid division may be more susceptible to chemicals that will result in genetic damage. This is why the sex hormone estrogen plays an important role in the development of breast cancer. The longer a woman's breast tissue is exposed to the monthly hormone changes associated with menstrual periods, the greater her risk of harmful genetic mutations. Women who begin having menstrual periods at an early age or continue to have them beyond the age of fifty-five are at somewhat greater risk of breast cancer. Risk is also

CAN MEN GET BREAST CANCER?

Yes, but rarely. Each year, about 1,500 men in the United States are diagnosed with breast cancer. Many men who develop symptoms are not aware that they can get breast cancer, or they may feel embarrassed about having a "woman's disease." When actor Richard Roundtree was diagnosed with breast cancer in 1993, he kept it secret from the public for six years. Since then, he has helped to educate men to be on the alert for breast cancer. Although very rare at any age, it occurs most frequently among men in their sixties.

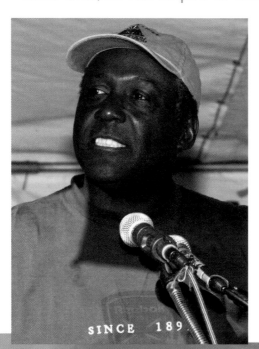

According to the American Cancer Society, 1,690 men will be diagnosed with breast cancer in 2005. Breast cancer survivor Richard Roundtree speaks at a breast cancer research walk in Santa Monica, California, in 2001. The survival rate for men is usually lower than for women, mainly because the cancer is often detected at a later stage.

higher among women who have never been pregnant or those who have a first child after the age of thirty. The discovery that childless women have a higher rate of breast cancer explains the observation made hundreds of years ago that the disease was more common among nuns, giving rise to its name "nun's disease." Recent research

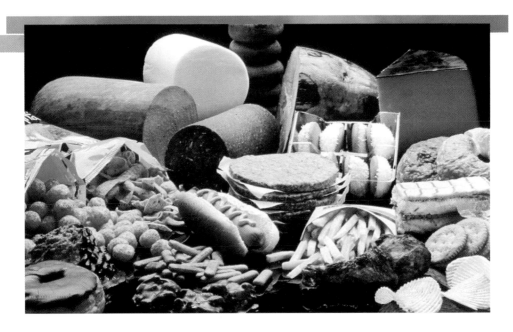

Above is a display of foods that belong to the saturated, or "bad," fats category. There is debate over how much a high-fat diet increases the risk of breast cancer. Unsaturated, or "good," fats include olive oil and nuts. However, obesity, which may result from a high-fat diet, is found to be a breast cancer risk.

also indicates an increase in breast cancer cases among women who take hormones as therapy for the symptoms of menopause.

Besides age, heredity, reproductive history, and hormone use, scientists have noted differences in numbers among ethnic groups. In the United States, breast cancer occurs more often in white women than among Latina, Asian, or African American women. Studies of women immigrants suggest that there is also an environmental component to the risk of breast cancer, as women of some ethnic backgrounds tend to develop the disease at a greater rate after they migrate to the United States. For example, although Japanese women have a low risk of breast cancer, those who migrate to the United States have been shown to have breast cancer rates similar to the general U.S. population within two generations of migration. Scientists cannot fully explain the increased cancer risk, but they think it may be related to changes in eating habits or substances in the environment.

Radiation of the breast at a young age and obesity in women after menopause are also related to higher breast cancer rates. Some studies have suggested that reduced physical activity, a high-fat diet, alcoholic beverages, and certain chemicals in the environment may be related to breast cancer rates. Scientists continue to study these and other complex issues surrounding the disease.

MYTHS ABOUT BREAST CANCER

Through the years, many theories about the causes of breast cancer have not held up under scientific investigation. In the early half of the twentieth century, magazines warned women that tight-fitting brassieres could lead to breast cancer. We now know this is false. Breast cancer cannot be caused by bumping or bruising the breasts, or by touching them. It is not possible to "catch" breast cancer from another person. Some have suggested an association between induced abortions and breast cancer. However, several extensive scientific studies have provided solid evidence that there is no association between abortion and breast cancer risk.

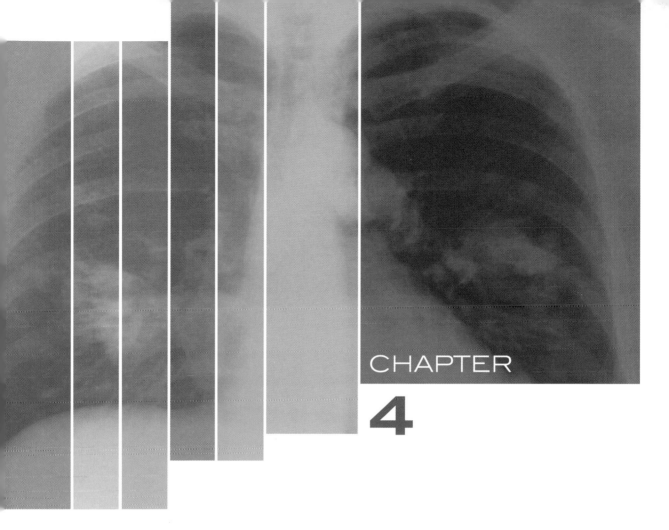

TREATMENT FOR BREAST CANCER

The world of breast cancer treatments is as complex as the disease itself. Women diagnosed with breast cancer must enter this world quickly, with little time to understand all the choices that confront them. Fortunately, many books, Web sites, cancer survivors, and health professionals are available to guide them. Standard treatments exist for some common forms of breast cancer, making decisions somewhat easier. It is not yet possible to be 100 percent sure which treatment is best in every case. Thus, a

THE CANCER THERAPY THAT ALMOST WASN'T

In the 1960s, a joint program of the National Cancer Institute (NCI) and the U.S. Department of Agriculture collected plant samples from all over the country as part of their search for effective anticancer therapies. One sample came from the bark of a scraggly tree in the Gifford Pinchot National Forest in Washington. The tree was a Pacific yew, *Taxus brevifolia*, a slow-growing tree found only in coastal areas of western states. The bark sample went through a laboratory screening process along with hundreds of other plant samples, and scientists were excited to find that the Pacific yew showed special toxic (cell-killing) properties.

Scientists clamored for more yew bark in order to study whether its toxic properties might work against cancer cells,

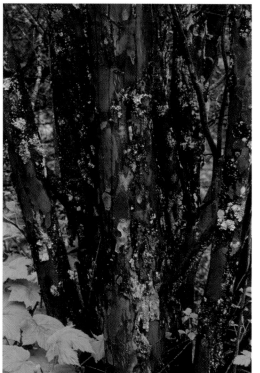

The Pacific yew is an evergreen. The one pictured here is located in Oregon. Taxol can be found in varying concentrations in all parts of the yew species tree. However, due to the small quantities in which it is found, it would take from three to ten trees per patient for treatment. Fortunately, Taxol can now be chemically synthesized.

but the NCI resisted because of the difficulty of obtaining it. Bark from a single tree could provide only a tiny amount of the chemical compound that the scientists wanted to test, and stripping the tree of its bark killed the tree. By coincidence, the forests where the trees were found were also part of various lawsuits filed by environmentalists trying to protect the habitat of the endangered spotted owl. This made any tree harvest a touchy issue.

For several years, yew bark research stayed "on the shelf" because of the supply problem. Finally, scientists were able to obtain enough bark to establish that the chemical extracted from it had anticancer activity. The scientists also learned that the compound had special properties different from other cancer drugs. It was given the name Taxol.

Early patient trials proved that Taxol would be an effective drug for treating cancer, but the supply problem remained. Soon all the yews in the western forests would be gone if they were stripped of bark to prepare a cancer drug. Finally, scientists figured out a way to synthesize the bark's important chemical compound. Hence, it was no longer necessary to harvest yew trees.

Taxol was approved by the U.S. Food and Drug Administration in 1992, more than twenty years after its discovery, and is now one of the most effective treatments for breast cancer. On July 10, 1999, the drug was among the emergency medical supplies airdropped at the South Pole, and was the first cancer treatment received by Dr. Jerri Nielsen (see introduction).

SYSTEMIC TREATMENT

Although local therapy remains an essential component of breast cancer therapy, emphasis in recent years has shifted to systemic therapy, as scientists have come to understand breast cancer as a systemic disease. Most tumors have existed for six to eight years prior to diagnosis, and there is a good chance that tumor cells have spread beyond the local tumor. Systemic therapies circulate through the bloodstream and can act on cancer cells wherever they occur in the body. This allows treatment of cancers that have spread to parts of the body distant from the breast tumor. Women generally receive systemic therapy in addition to local therapy, even if no tumors can be detected, in case cancer cells have already spread beyond the tumor site. When women with no evidence of cancer receive systemic therapy following local therapy, it is called adjuvant therapy.

Systemic therapies fall into three major types: chemotherapy, hormonal therapy, and biological therapy. A systemic treatment regimen usually consists of a combination of agents from one or more of these types. A combination of therapies is used because it is not possible to be sure which type of therapy will kill the cells of a particular tumor. Also, some tumor cells may change over time and a single tumor may contain a mixture of cells, each killed by a different therapy. When tumor cells are killed by therapy, or stopped from growing, doctors say that the tumor is "responding" to that therapy. If a tumor does not respond to a therapy, or if it comes back after treatment, physicians will usually suggest switching to a different therapy to see if the tumor will respond.

CHEMOTHERAPY

A cancer chemotherapy is a toxic chemical that can kill cells when they are in the process of division. Different chemotherapies interfere with the cell division process in different ways, so some tumor cells will be

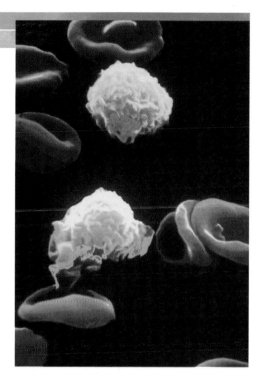

Red and white blood cells are pictured here. A decrease of these rapidly dividing cells is a side effect of chemotherapy. A decrease in red blood cells can result in anemia, when body tissues do not get enough oxygen to function normally. Symptoms include fatigue, paleness, or dizziness. A decrease in white blood cells is called leukopenia, and the risk of infection is increased. Chemotherapy patients are closely monitored for these side effects.

killed by certain chemotherapies and not by others. Since not all cancer cells are dividing at any one time, chemotherapy treatments are repeated for several weeks or months. If the chemotherapy is effective, the number of cancer cells is gradually reduced until the amount is small enough for the body's immune system to eliminate the rest.

A drawback to chemotherapy is that it can kill any dividing cells, not just cancer cells. Cells in the bone marrow are constantly dividing to produce red blood cells, white blood cells, and platelets. When a woman is receiving chemotherapy, her doctor will monitor the level of these blood cells to be sure they do not get too low. A common problem is the development of infections, such as pneumonia, because there are not enough white blood cells to fight disease. Hair cells also divide rapidly. These may be killed by chemotherapy, which is why many people lose their hair while receiving chemotherapy. Hair grows back once chemotherapy is stopped.

HORMONAL THERAPY

When a woman undergoes surgery to remove a breast tumor, some tissue from the tumor is tested to see if the cells have hormone receptors. If so, and about two-thirds of tumors do, the tumor is said to be hormone receptor positive, or ER-positive ("ER" for "estrogen"). An ER-positive tumor will probably respond to hormonal therapy. Some hormonal therapies work by lowering the body's supply of estrogen— without estrogen, these tumor cells will not continue to divide. This may be accomplished in some cases by surgical removal of a woman's ovaries in order to eliminate a source of estrogen production, or by administering drugs that suppress estrogen production. Another hormonal approach is to change the body's hormonal environment so that estrogen cannot interact with the cancer cells. One very effective hormonal therapy, tamoxifen, blocks the tumor's hormone receptors. Although scientists still do not understand the process completely, it seems that over a long period of exposure to tamoxifen, the tumor cells are no longer active. Most women with ER-positive tumors are treated with hormonal therapy for several years after their cancer surgery. Since hormonal therapy acts only on certain types of cells rather than on all dividing cells, there are fewer side effects compared to chemotherapy.

BIOLOGICAL THERAPY

Certain newer cancer therapies are referred to as biological therapies because they take advantage of biological properties of a particular tumor. Scientists who study breast cancer cells at the molecular level try to find out what has gone wrong in the normal cell processes to change them to tumor cells. When they find something abnormal, they try to find a chemical that can interfere with the abnormality and make the cells die. It is much more difficult than it might seem to find a new biological therapy, and so far only one such therapy is effective in treating breast cancer.

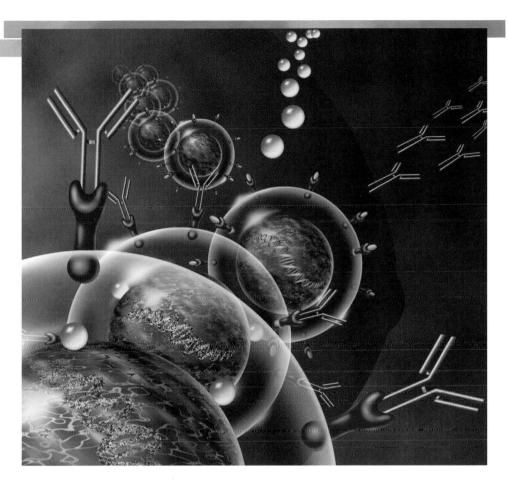

This is an illustration of how the antibody herceptin (the "Y" shaped objects) binds with the receptors on the cell's surface (in red) where the HER-2 gene is activated in order to prevent tumor cell proliferation. Chemotherapy is represented by the green spheres.

Herceptin is a biological therapy that can kill breast cancer cells with activation of the HER-2 gene, which we learned about in chapter 2. Biological therapies have a big advantage compared to chemotherapy: side effects are minimal since they target only the cancer cells.

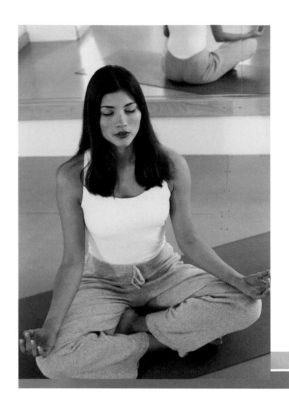

This woman is in a meditation pose, as part of her yoga practice. Yoga is a Sanskrit word meaning "union." It integrates movement, breathing, and meditation to achieve a state of relaxation. Although it is not a treatment for cancer, it is believed to relieve stress that can be present during the time of cancer treatment. As some poses can be quite rigorous and possibly stressful to certain muscle groups and joints, breast cancer patients are advised to consult their physicians before starting this complementary therapy.

COMPLEMENTARY AND ALTERNATIVE TREATMENT

Some women with breast cancer have sought help from complementary or alternative therapies. Alternative therapies are those used to treat cancer in place of the usual therapies described earlier, and include such things as herbal mixtures and special diets. None of these has been found effective for treatment of cancer. Complementary therapies are those used to supplement usual therapies, and include meditation, counseling, prayer, yoga, acupuncture, and diet supplements. These may help a woman feel better while she is receiving other therapy.

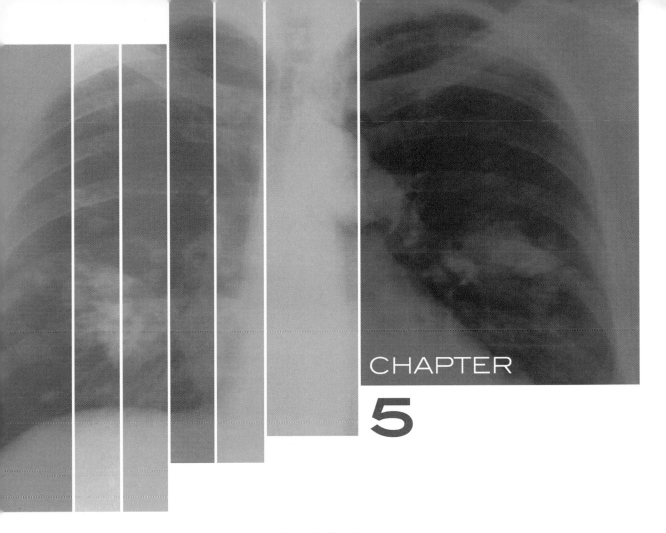

CAN WE PREVENT BREAST CANCER?

Breast cancer researchers would like nothing better than to find a way to prevent breast cancer. It is not a reality yet, but today's young women will benefit from studies now under way. Many of these studies focus on chemoprevention: a woman would perhaps take a daily pill that would reduce her risk of getting breast cancer. Additional research looks for tests that will tell which women are at high risk of getting breast cancer and would thus benefit most from prevention strategies.

CHEMOPREVENTION

One drug, tamoxifen, has been shown to reduce the risk of getting breast cancer in certain groups of women. It is the same drug used to treat women who already have breast cancer. Before a cancer develops, a normal cell must undergo a series of changes in its genetic material, or mutations, as described in chapter 2. If a cell divides that has experienced only the first of these mutations, there are more "precancer" cells that have a chance of undergoing further mutations and changing into cancer cells. Since estrogen can encourage breast cell division, it may increase the chance that a precancer cell will become cancerous. Researchers had the idea that giving tamoxifen, which blocks the estrogen effect, would decrease the risk of breast cancer. When they tested this idea in a study of thousands of women, they found fewer cases of breast cancer among the women who took tamoxifen compared to those who took a similar-looking pill that contained no drug. However, some undesirable side effects may occur when taking the drug, so doctors only recommend it for women who have a high chance of getting breast cancer.

LIFESTYLE CHANGES

The risk of breast cancer may be reduced by certain lifestyle changes, though researchers are less sure about their specific effects. Some studies show that women who exercise regularly, who follow a healthy diet and are not obese, and who do not drink alcohol are less apt to develop breast cancer. A large randomized trial in 2002 showed that women taking hormones for treatment of menopause symptoms were more likely to develop breast cancer. Women with menopause symptoms must now carefully consider whether the benefits of hormone replacement therapy are worth the possible increased risk of breast cancer.

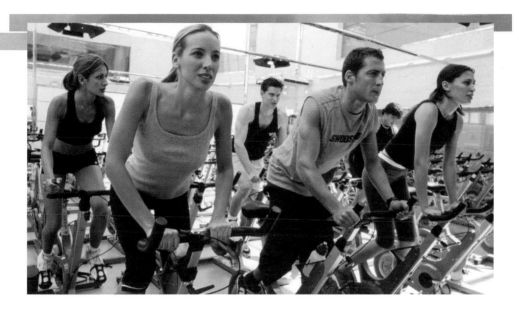

Keeping fit has numerous benefits, and various studies show that regular exercise and physical activity may protect both pre- and postmenopausal women from the risk of breast cancer. This is because regular exercise decreases estrogen levels. Even low- to moderate-impact exercise can boost the immune system and help the body kill cancer cells or slow their growth rate.

SURGERY

An approach to prevention that is rarely used is the surgical removal of both breasts. This drastic approach is considered only for women who are at high risk of breast cancer because of their family history and who are very concerned about the possibility of getting breast cancer.

EARLY DETECTION OF BREAST CANCER

Since we cannot yet prevent breast cancer, the next best strategy is to find the cancers when they are very small and probably curable. This process, called screening, involves frequent checking for evidence of

WHY ISN'T MAMMOGRAPHY GOOD ENOUGH?

About eight of one hundred screening mammograms find an abnormality in the breast. An abnormal mammogram may cause the woman involved to be very anxious. Yet the woman is found to have breast cancer in fewer than 10 percent of these cases. When a mammogram is abnormal and a woman does not have cancer, it is called "false-positive." A test with a high false-positive rate is not a very good test. In about one of four cases of abnormal mammograms, a woman must undergo a biopsy—a procedure that has some side effects and is costly for the medical system. A further drawback is that mammograms detect some precancers that might never become

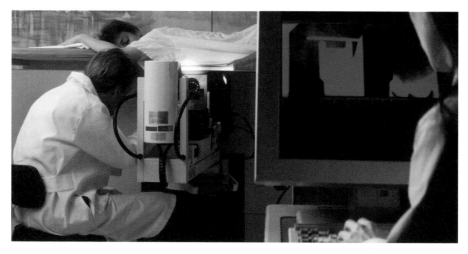

This woman is having a stereotactic biopsy performed. In this procedure, the patient lies facedown on a specialized table. The breast is compressed through an opening, much like a mammogram. The radiologist uses both ultrasound and mammography to help with accurately inserting the needle in lesions deep within the breast tissue. A tiny metallic marker can be left at the site to monitor the irregularity in future mammograms.

cancers, or very slowly growing cancers. A woman with one of these conditions could live a full lifespan never knowing or worrying about breast cancer. Still, once it is detected on a mammogram, the woman and her doctors will probably decide that it must be treated since there is no way to be certain it is harmless. Mammograms may also miss some cases of cancer. These drawbacks have researchers seeking better methods to detect breast cancers early and to develop tests with low false-positive rates.

cancer. The most important screening test for breast cancer is called mammography. In mammography, a trained technician uses a low-dose X-ray machine to take a picture of the tissues inside the breast. Physicians with special training in diagnosis procedures can look at these pictures to see if there is any sign of cancer. If an abnormality is found, a woman will have additional testing to find out if cancer is present.

The National Cancer Institute recommends that women older than forty have a mammogram every one or two years. Studies have shown that having regular mammograms reduces a woman's chance of dying from breast cancer. Still, there are some drawbacks to their use, and women whose cancers are detected by mammography may still die of breast cancer. The average size of a tumor detected by mammography repeated at recommended intervals is only one-eighth of an inch (three-tenths of a centimeter)—too small to be felt by breast examination.

In addition to mammograms, women should have annual examinations of their breasts by their health-care providers. Many health professionals recommend that women examine their own breasts for lumps every month, although there is no real evidence that this practice reduces breast cancer deaths.

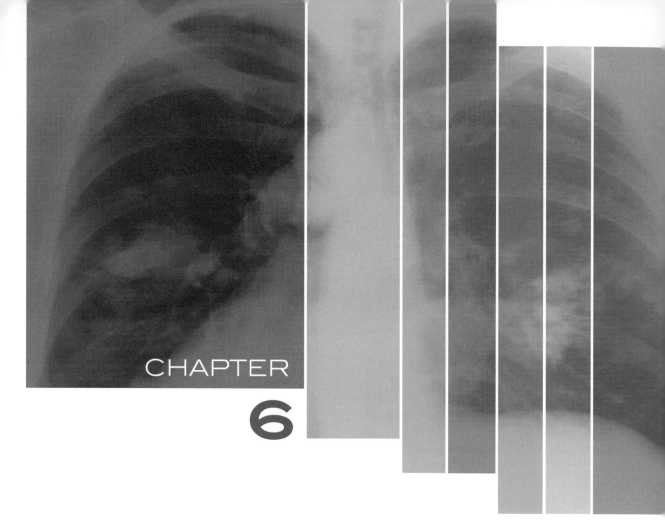

CHAPTER

6

THE PROMISE OF RESEARCH

Cancer researchers around the world are following exciting leads that will bring about improvements in breast cancer prevention, diagnosis, and treatment. Physicians, technicians, molecular biologists, computer experts, biochemists, geneticists, statisticians, nurses, epidemiologists, and others are all working together to answer complicated scientific questions about breast cancer. They are making rapid progress, especially in understanding how disease processes work at the molecular level within cancer cells.

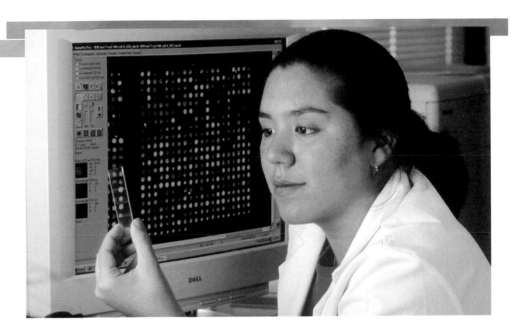

DNA microarray technology allows scientists to look at numerous genes at once and determine which are being expressed in a particular type of cell or tissue. This lab technician is holding a microscope slide on which DNA molecules are placed. Thousands of genes can be present on a single slide. This technology can produce precise, critical information about the molecular makeup of a tumor cell.

MOLECULAR TECHNOLOGY

Each human cell is estimated to contain about 30,000 genes. In every type of normal body tissue, only a limited number of these genes within the cells are active, or "switched on," with different genes switched on depending on the type of tissue. When a gene is active within a cell, it directs the production of proteins that carry out the body's functions. In the cancer process, genetic mutations cause different genes to be switched on or off compared to normal cells, and these changes in genes lead to production of different proteins as well. Scientists have

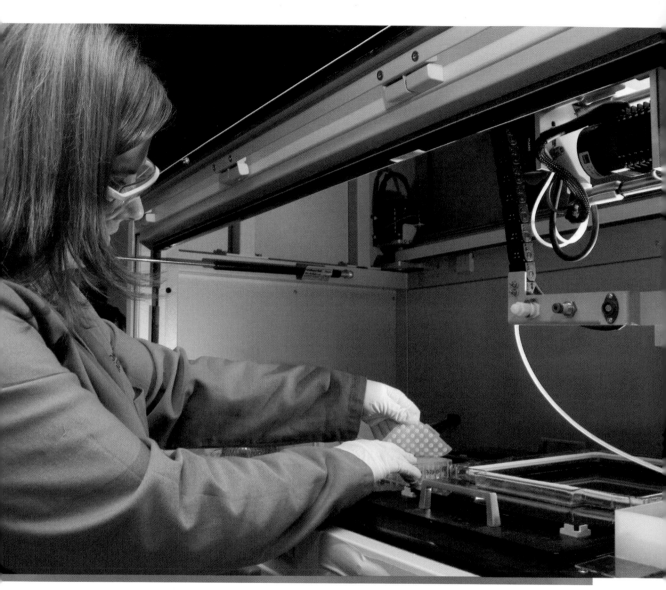

Whereas the entire human genome of 30,000 genes has been sequenced, only a small percentage of the 1 to 10 million proteins found in human cells has been identified. Yet protein identification may be a promising lead to cancer prevention, screening, and treatment. This researcher is picking proteins for identification.

powerful new tools available to help them understand and measure these processes. Microarray technology allows scientists to simultaneously measure several thousand genes in a tissue sample from a breast tumor to determine if the genes are switched on or off. Similarly, the new technology of proteomics allows the study of thousands of proteins, which are produced by genes within the cells of a tumor. By applying these methods to a tumor sample from a woman with breast cancer, scientists hope they can determine what has gone wrong in the genetic material that caused the cells to become cancerous. This may give doctors the information they need to decide the best treatment for that woman. If it turns out that certain genes are abnormal in almost every woman with breast cancer, researchers may be able to devise a test to find that abnormal gene in healthy women, before it causes cancer, or find treatments that will correct the abnormal gene. These abnormal genes or proteins are referred to as tumor biomarkers. Hundreds of them are being investigated already and more will doubtlessly be discovered. Each one is given a coded name such as HER-2, p53, and cyclin E.

An example of success in using this molecular information is the systemic drug Herceptin (see chapter 4), which scientists developed after they discovered the abnormal HER-2 gene. Only about a third of breast cancers have this abnormal gene, however, and even when it is present, some tumors do not respond. Each tumor is complex, containing a mixture of cells, not all of which may be affected by Herceptin. If too many unaffected cells continue to grow, the treatment will not be effective.

As research uncovers more tumor biomarkers, scientists work to find drugs that will act against the specific genetic abnormalities indicated by the biomarkers. Their hope is that a woman's tumor may one day be thought of as having a "barcode," just like items at the grocery store. Once the abnormal genes for that particular tumor are identified in the barcode, the woman will receive a combination of treatments that will target and kill all the cells of her tumor. It may even be possible to find certain biomarkers to identify tumors that are not capable of spreading beyond the breast. In this case, a woman would be cured by local therapy and she would not need to receive any further therapy. Now, almost every woman with breast cancer must receive systemic chemotherapy because her physician cannot be sure if a particular tumor is able to spread.

ADVANCES IN LOCAL THERAPY

Scientists are conducting research aimed at reducing the duration and side effects of treatment. For example, when surgeons remove the armpit lymph nodes during breast cancer surgery, women may have problems with swelling in the arm, and there may be nerve damage. In a new procedure, surgeons identify an important lymph node, called the sentinel node. If there are no cancer cells in this node, the surgeon can be sure that the armpit nodes do not contain cancer and it is safe to

COULD ASPIRIN PREVENT BREAST CANCER?

Scientific literature provides growing evidence that taking aspirin (or similar nonsteroidal anti-inflammatory drugs) may be effective in preventing breast cancer. In a study of 1,442 women with breast cancer and 1,420 women who did not have breast cancer, researchers found that women without breast cancer were more likely to have been frequent users of aspirin prior to the study, compared to the women who had breast cancer. Still, the difference was fairly small, and researchers cannot be sure that the aspirin prevented cases of breast cancer. This is just one of many such leads researchers are following as they look for ways to prevent breast cancer.

leave them. Surgeons are studying a method to destroy tumors with heat by putting tiny electrodes through the skin of the breast. If this method works, some women with breast cancer may not even have to undergo surgery. New techniques being studied for the administration of radiotherapy may greatly reduce the standard time of four to six weeks of treatment.

IMPROVED METHODS OF CANCER DETECTION

At least one type of cancer can now be detected by testing a blood sample. If such a test could be discovered for breast cancer, this would be much better than mammograms, which are inconvenient for women, detect many false-positive cases, and require expensive equipment. Scientists think that breast cancer cells release biomarker proteins into the bloodstream. They hope to use proteomic technology to find a protein that is in the blood of women with breast cancer, but does not occur in women without breast cancer. This would lead to a cheap and effective test that women might be able to get on a trip to the shopping mall. It would identify only those women very likely to have cancer, in contrast to mammograms, which find many noncancer abnormalities as well.

Other scientists are working on tests of cells that they remove from a woman's breast ducts. If these tests show abnormalities in the breast cells of women who have not been diagnosed with breast cancer, it might lead to methods to diagnose very early cancers or to identify women at high risk of developing cancer.

RESEARCH IN PREVENTING BREAST CANCER

Just as the new understanding of cancer at the molecular level can lead to successful treatment, it is possible to apply this knowledge at an even earlier stage of the developing cancer so that it can be prevented from

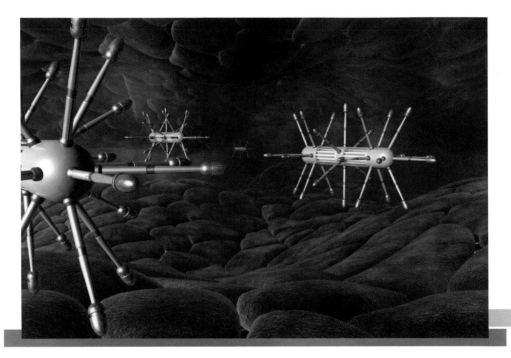

This artist's illustration depicts how nanotechnology may be used in the future to treat diseases from within the human body. Presently, however, nanotechnology consists of nanoparticles. These bits are being experimented on to take on different capabilities. One type of research to treat cancer involves hollow spheres of gold or silver "shells" that would be injected into a tumor. The hollowness would allow the nanoparticles to heat up when an infrared light is shined on them. These heated particles then kill the tumor.

becoming a tumor at all. We already know that the cancer process begins because something is wrong in the genetic material of a person. Once this genetic error is present, other influences control whether it leads to a cancer. There may be certain chemicals in our environment, or in our bodies, that cause further genetic changes that lead to cancer. Researchers hope to use molecular technology to identify chemicals that cause these changes or that promote the growth of cancer cells.

Scientists must first understand more about the complex interactions of genetic damage and substances such as hormones and environmental chemicals. These substances can act to promote cancer in the presence of genetic damage. Then, there will be enormous opportunities for finding ways to prevent breast cancer.

NANOTECHNOLOGY

The new science of nanotechnology involves working with very tiny particles (about 1/80,000th the width of a human hair) to develop devices that researchers hope can be used for the prevention, diagnosis, and treatment of cancer. Scientists are just beginning to learn how such tiny devices can be manipulated, and how they can be put to use within the human body. For example, it may be possible to design a device with a tiny hole just large enough for a strand of genetic material to pass through for examination. If an error is found, this could help researchers understand the genetic process leading to cancer.

PROGRESS CONTINUES

As we think back to the methods used to treat breast cancer in past centuries, and the unfortunate women who suffered at the hands of well-meaning but ill-informed physicians, we recognize that tremendous progress has been made. Women diagnosed with breast cancer today can seek help from highly skilled professionals. They can have a reasonable expectation that their disease will be cured. However, scientists realize that there is still much they do not understand about the disease. As scientists continue to make progress against the disease on many fronts, we may hope that women someday will have nothing to fear if they should find a lump in their breast.

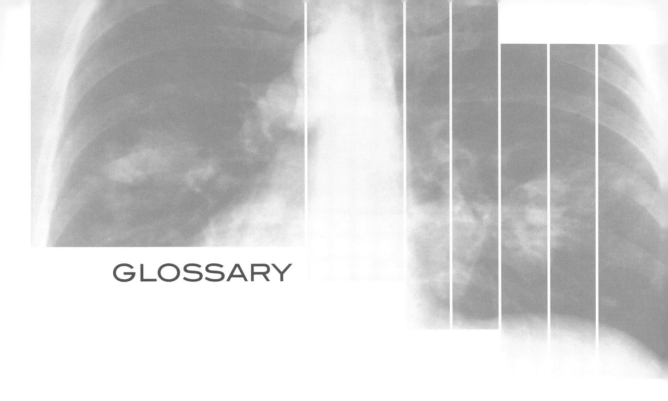

GLOSSARY

adjuvant therapy Anticancer drugs given before there is a detectable spread of cancer beyond the breast area; used in combination with local therapy to prevent recurrence.

axilla Armpit or area under the arm.

biomarker Substance found in the blood, cancer cells, or elsewhere, which may indicate a certain type of cancer if it occurs at abnormal levels; also called tumor marker.

BRCA1, BRCA2 Genes associated with a higher risk of breast cancer when abnormal.

complementary therapy Practices used in addition to standard treatment for a disease; often aimed at improving a patient's quality of life.

DNA Deoxyribonucleic acid; a series of chemicals in the cell nucleus that make up the body's genetic code.

HER-2 gene Gene that produces the HER-2 protein that is involved in growth of some cancer cells.

hormone receptor Location on cell surface to which hormone molecules can attach.

lobe A portion of an organ.

lobule A subdivision of a lobe; in the breast, the part that is able to produce milk.

local treatment Treatment that affects only the tumor and nearby tissue.

menopause Time when a woman's menstrual periods stop permanently, usually around age fifty.

randomized study Study in which the treatment for a participant is decided at random (like the flip of a coin) from among two or more such treatments; this assures comparability of treatment groups, allowing researchers to draw conclusions about which is the better treatment.

sentinel node First lymph node to which cancer cells from a breast tumor are likely to spread.

side effect Problem that occurs when a treatment affects other parts of the body rather than what it is meant to treat; examples of chemotherapy side effects are nausea and hair loss.

systemic treatment Treatment that travels through the bloodstream and reaches the whole body.

tamoxifen Treatment able to block the effect of estrogen; used in prevention and treatment of breast cancer.

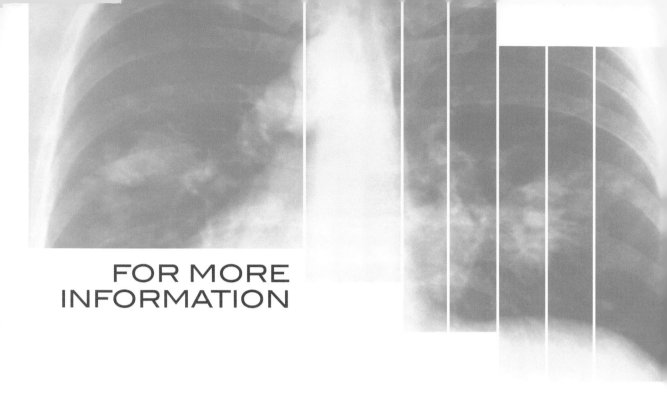

FOR MORE INFORMATION

American Cancer Society
15999 Clifton Road, NE
Atlanta, GA 30329-4251
(800) 227-2345
Web site: http://www.cancer.org

FORCE: Facing Our Risk of Cancer Empowered
16057 Tampa Palms Boulevard W., PMB #373
Tampa, FL 33647
(954) 255-8732
Web site: http://www.facingourrisk.org

Imaginis Corp., The Women's Health Resource
P.O. Box 27018
Greenville, SC 29616
e-mail: learnmore@imaginis.com
Web site: http://www.imaginis.com

MEDLINEplus
U.S. National Library of Medicine
8600 Rockville Pike
Bethesda, MD 20894
Web site: http://www.nlm.nih.gov/medlineplus

National Breast Cancer Coalition
1707 L Street NW, Suite 1060
Washington, DC 20036
(202) 296-7477
Web site: http://www.natlbcc.org

National Cancer Institute
31 Center Drive, MSC 2580
Bethesda, MD 20892-2580
Cancer Information Service (800) 4-CANCER [(800) 422-6237]
Web site: http://www.cancer.gov

OncoLink
University of Pennsylvania Medical Center
3400 Spruce Street—2 Donner
Philadelphia, PA 19104
Web site: http://www.oncolink.upenn.edu/disease/breast

Susan G. Komen Breast Cancer Foundation
5005 LBJ Freeway, Suite 250
Dallas, TX 75244
(972) 855-1600
Web site: http://www.komen.org

SusanLoveMD.org
P.O. Box 846
Pacific Palisades, CA 90272
(310) 230-1712
Web site: http://www.susanlovemd.org

University of Texas M.D. Anderson Cancer Center
1515 Holcombe Boulevard
Houston, TX 77030
(800) 392-1611
Web site: http://www.mdanderson.org/care_centers/breastcenter

IN CANADA
Breast Cancer Society of Canada
125 Michigan Avenue
Point Edward, ON N7V 1E5
Canada
(800) 567-8767
e-mail: bcsc@bcsc.ca
Web site: http://www.bcsc.ca

Canadian Breast Cancer Foundation
790 Bay Street, Suite 1000
Toronto, ON M5G 1N8
Canada
(800) 387-9816
e-mail: cbcf@cbcf.org
Web site: http://www.cbcf.org

National Cancer Institute of Canada
10 Alcorn Avenue, Suite 200
Toronto, ON M4V 3B1
Canada
416-961-7223
e-mail: ncic@cancer.ca
Web site: http://www.ncic.ca

WEB SITES

Due to the changing nature of Internet links, the Rosen Publishing Group, Inc., has developed an online list of Web sites related to the subject of this book. This site is updated regularly. Please use this link to access the list:

http://www.rosenlinks.com/cms/brca

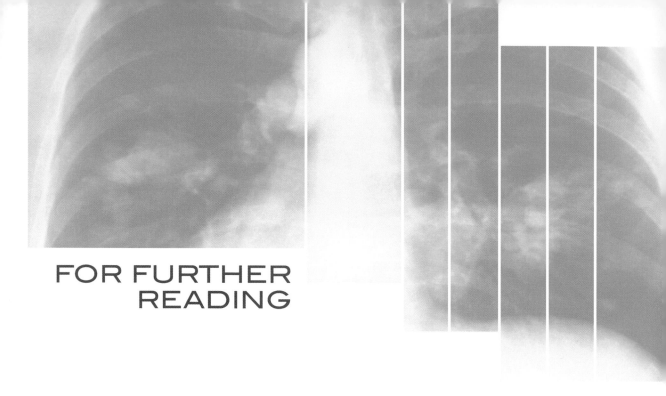

FOR FURTHER READING

Eisenpreis, Bettijane. *A Young Woman's Guide to Breast Cancer Prevention*. New York, NY: Rosen Publishing Group, Inc., 1999.

Love, Susan M. *Dr. Susan Love's Breast Book*, 3rd ed. Cambridge, MA: Perseus Publishing, 2000.

Majure, Janet. *Diseases and People: Breast Cancer*. Berkeley Heights, NJ: Enslow Publishers, Inc., 2000.

National Cancer Institute, National Institutes of Health. *What You Need to Know About Breast Cancer*, NIH Publication No. 03-1556. Washington, DC: National Institutes of Health, 2003.

Nielsen, Jerri. *Icebound. A Doctor's Incredible Battle for Survival at the South Pole.* New York, NY: Hyperion, 2001.

Olson, James S. *Bathsheba's Breast: Women, Cancer & History*. Baltimore, MD: Johns Hopkins University Press, 2002.

Pfeuffer, Charyn. *Breast Cancer Q & A: Insightful Answers to the 100 Most Frequently Asked Questions*. New York, NY: Avery, 2003.

Vogel, Carole G. *Breast Cancer: Questions & Answers for Young Women*. Brookfield, CT: Twenty-first Century Books, 2001.

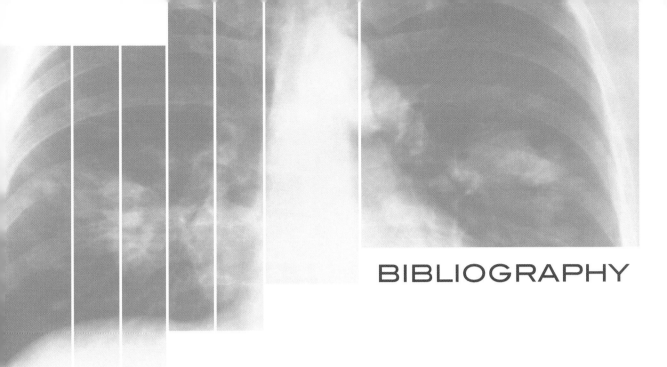

BIBLIOGRAPHY

Berry, D. A., T. L. Smith, and A. U. Buzdar. "Breast Cancer." *Textbook of Clinical Trials*. Edited by David Machin, Simon Day, and Sylvan Green. Hoboken, NJ: John Wiley & Sons, 2004.

Buchanan, Edwin B. "A Century of Breast Cancer Surgery." *Cancer Investigation*, Vol. 14, No. 1, 1996, pp. 371 377.

Esteva, F., G. Hortobaygi, A. Sahin, T. L. Smith, D. Chin, S-Y. Liang, L. Pusztai, A. Buzdar, and S. Bacus "Expression of erbB/HER Receptors, Heregulin and P38 in Primary Breast Cancer Using Quantitative Immunohistochemistry." *Pathology Oncology Research*, Vol. 7, 2001, pp. 171–177.

Fisher, Bernard. "Personal Contributions to Progress in Breast Cancer Research and Treatment." *Seminars in Oncology*, Vol. 23, No. 4, 1996, pp. 414–427.

Fisher, B., J. P. Costantino, D. L. Wickerham, et al. "Tamoxifen for Prevention of Breast Cancer: Report of the National Surgical Adjuvant Breast and Bowel Project P-1 Study." *Journal of the National Cancer Institute*, Vol. 90, No. 18, 1998, pp. 1371–88.

Giordano, S. H., A. U. Buzdar, T. L. Smith, S. W. Kau, Y. Yang, and G. N. Hortogagyi. "Is Breast Cancer Survival Improving?" *Cancer*, Vol. 100, No. 1, 2004, pp. 44–52.

Kaspar, Anne S., and Susan J. Ferguson, eds. *Breast Cancer: Society Shapes an Epidemic*. New York, NY: St. Martin's Press, 2000.

Leyland-Jones, Brian, and Ian Smith. "Role of Herceptin in Primary Breast Cancer: Views from North America and Europe." *Oncology*, Vol. 61, Suppl. 2, 2001, pp. 83–91.

Love, Susan M. *Dr. Susan Love's Breast Book,* 3rd ed. Cambridge, MA: Perseus Publishing, 2000.

National Cancer Institute. "Breast Cancer (PDQ): Treatment." Retrieved October 4, 2004 (http://www.cancer.gov/cancerinfo/pdq/treatment/breast/patient).

National Cancer Institute. "Male Breast Cancer (PDQ): Treatment." Retrieved October 4, 2004 (http://www.cancer.gov/cancerinfo/pdq/treatment/malebreast/patient).

National Cancer Institute. "Science Behind the News." Retrieved October 4, 2004 (http://press2.nci.nih.gov/sciencebehind/index.htm).

Nielsen, Jerri. *Icebound. A Doctor's Incredible Battle for Survival at the South Pole.* New York, NY: Hyperion, 2001.

Olson, James S. *Bathsheba's Breast. Women, Cancer & History*. Baltimore, MD: Johns Hopkins University Press, 2002.

Singletary, S. E., C. Allred, P. Ashley, et al. "Revision of the American Joint Committee on Cancer Staging System for Breast Cancer." *Journal of Clinical Oncology*, Vol. 20, 2002, pp. 3628–3636.

Terry, M. B., M. D. Gammon, F. F. Zhang, et al. "Association of Frequency and Duration of Aspirin Use and Hormone Receptor Status with Breast Cancer Risk. *Journal of the American Medical Association*, Vol. 291, No. 20, 2004, pp. 2433–2440.

Wall, Monroe E., and Mansukh C. Wani. "Camptothecin and Taxol: From Discovery to Clinic." *Journal of Ethnopharmacology*, Vol. 51, 1996, pp. 239–254.

Writing Group for the Women's Health Initiative Investigators. "Risks and Benefits of Estrogen Plus Progestin in Healthy Postmenopausal Women: Principal Results from the Women's Health Initiative Randomized Controlled Trial." *Journal of the American Medical Association*, Vol. 288, No. 3, 2002, pp. 321–333.

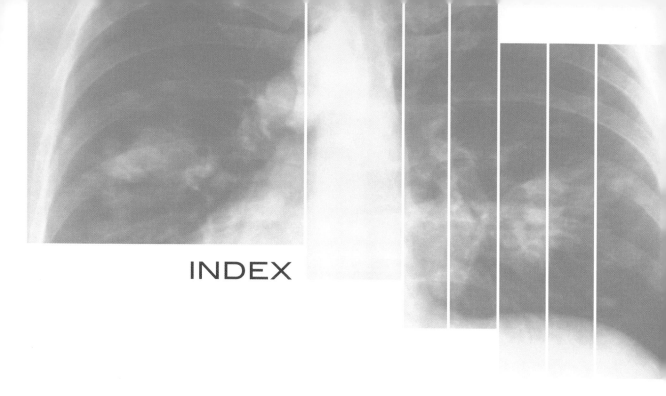

INDEX

ABOUT THE AUTHOR
Terry L. Smith, M.S., is a statistician and science writer living in Santa Fe, New Mexico. She formerly served on the faculty of the University of Texas M. D. Anderson Cancer Center in Houston, Texas, and is a coauthor of more than 200 scientific articles about cancer.

PHOTO CREDITS